Anti Aging Beginners Guide

Home practical steps to engage in, with no age limits. Get the secrets to achieving your desired look

Bonus: 30 days skin care routine for you

Eve C. Bird

Acknowledgement

Writing "Anti-Aging for Beginners Guide" has been a fantastic experience, and I am grateful to everyone who has encouraged and inspired me along the road.

First and foremost, I'd like to convey my heartfelt gratitude to the pioneers in the fields of health, fitness, and skincare whose innovative work has deeply shaped my understanding and viewpoint. To Dr. Nicholas Perricone, for his groundbreaking research into the anti-inflammatory diet and its astonishing effects on aging. Dr. David Sinclair, whose study on longevity and sirtuins has expanded horizons and motivated numerous people, including myself, to investigate the possibility of extending a healthy life. To Dr. Andrew Weil, whose holistic approach to health and well-being has taught me the value of balance in all aspects of life. Your contributions have been critical in shaping the book.

A particular thank you to my family, whose continuous support and encouragement have been my rock throughout this journey. Thank you, Francis, for your endless tolerance, love, and belief in my vision. Your messages of support and understanding during the long nights of writing meant more to me than I can say. My children, your curiosity and excitement for learning about health and wellbeing have been an ongoing source of inspiration. Every day, you remind me how vital it is to live a healthier, more vibrant life.

Finally, I'd like to thank my readers for joining me on this adventure. I sincerely hope that this book will be a great resource and source of inspiration for you as you embark on your own journey to a better, more fulfilled life.

With appreciation,

Eve C. Bird

Copyright

Eve C. Bird, 2024. Reserved rights apply. Without the author's explicit written consent, no portion of this book may be copied, stored in a retrieval system, or transmitted in any way, with the exception of condensed quotations used in reviews or critical articles.

Disclaimer

This book contains information solely for general informational purposes; it is not intended to be used as professional advice. The information provided here may be used or misused, and neither the publisher nor the author shall be held responsible for any results. In certain instances, it is advised to consult with a certified specialist.

About the Author

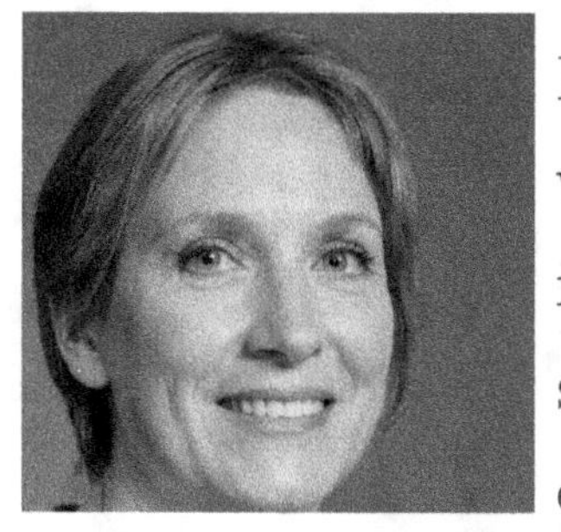

Eve C. Bird is a well-known authority in the fields of skincare, dietetics, exercise, and health. She is passionate about enabling people to live healthy, balanced lifestyles. She has become a reliable voice in the quest for holistic well-being because of her vast expertise gained from in-depth research and real-world experience. Her devotion to disseminating practical knowledge has positively impacted many lives and established a community of people committed to adopting a better, healthier way of living. Readers learn the transformative power of conscious decisions and uncover the keys to glowing health and revitalized skin with the help of Eve C. Bird.

How to use this book

Welcome to the "Anti-Aging for Beginners Guide"! This book is intended to be your full guide to adopting an anti-aging lifestyle, complete with practical advice, simple actions, and tangible results. To make the most of this guide, here's an easy way to navigate and use the content:

1. **Begin with the basics:** Begin with the introductory chapters to learn about the fundamentals of aging and how it affects the body. These parts serve as a solid foundation and background for the remainder of the book.

2. **Refer to the Step-by-Step Guide:** Each chapter is designed to build on the preceding one, providing a step-by-step

guide for adopting anti-aging activities into your daily routine.

- Chapter 1: Understand the science of aging and why it happens.
- Chapter 2: Learn the value of a healthy diet and regular exercise in maintaining youthfulness.
- Chapter 3: Discover efficient skincare practices to keep your skin healthy and shining.
- Chapter 4: Learn stress management skills to improve your mental health.
- Chapter 5: Recognize the importance of quality sleep in the aging process.
- Chapter 6:Explore the mind-body link via disciplines such as meditation and mindfulness.

- In Chapter 7, you'll learn about supplements that can help with anti-aging.

3. Implement the 30-Day Skincare Routine: Start your anti-aging skincare program with the precise 30-day routine provided. Follow the morning and night routines to notice visible results.

4. Customize Your Journey: This book invites you to adapt the recommendations to your specific needs. Pay attention to how your body reacts to certain practices and modify accordingly. The idea is to figure out what works best for you.

5. Use the resources: Throughout the book, you'll find useful suggestions, examples, and advice. Use these resources to design your own plan. To strengthen your understanding, each chapter may conclude with summaries or important takeaways.

6. Reflection and Progress: Keep a notebook to document your progress, noting any improvements in your health, appearance, and overall well-being. Reflection aids in understanding what works and maintaining motivation.

7. Join the community: Connect with other readers and share your experiences. Connecting with people, whether via social media or local groups, may bring both support and motivation.

This book is more than just a guide to a better, more vibrant life. Accept the process, remain consistent, and enjoy the path to achieving timeless vitality.

Best wishes for your health and happiness.

Bonus: 30-Day Skincare Routine

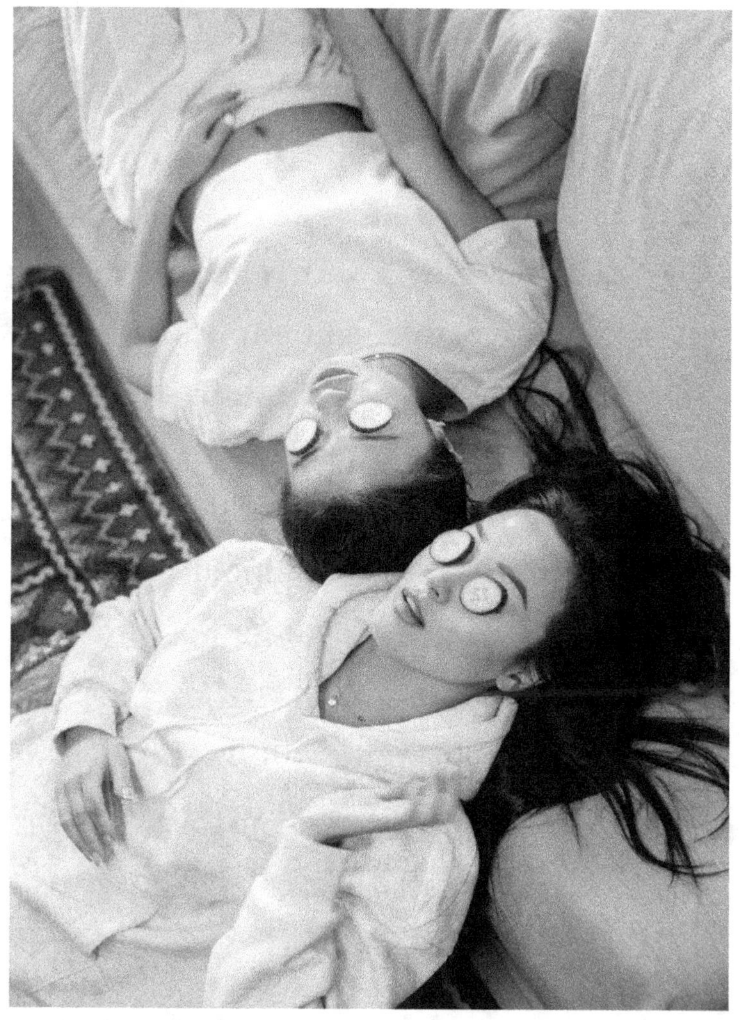

All the steps on how to choose the right products, what to look out for, and what to avoid are in this book.

Morning Routine:

Day 1-5:
- Cleanser: Begin with a gentle cleanser to remove overnight impurities.
- Toner: Apply a soothing toner to balance your skin's pH.
- Vitamin C Serum: Introduce vitamin C serum for a burst of antioxidants.
- Moisturizer: Hydrate with a lightweight moisturizer.
- SPF: Always finish with a broad-spectrum SPF to protect your skin.

Day 6-10:

- Cleanser
- Toner
- Serum: Include a specialized serum targeting specific skin concerns.
- Moisturizer
- SPF

Day 11-15:

- Cleanser
- Toner
- Vitamin C Serum
- Face Oil: Add a nourishing face oil for extra hydration.
- Moisturizer
- SPF

Night Routine:

Day 16-20:

- Cleanser: Opt for a cleanser that addresses nighttime build-up.
- Toner
- Serum: Use a targeted serum for evening skin repair.
- Moisturizer
- Eye Care: Apply an eye cream to hydrate and reduce puffiness.

Day 21-25:

- Cleanser
- Toner
- Retinol: Introduce retinol for skin renewal and rejuvenation.
- Moisturizer
- Eye Care

Day 26-30:

- Cleanser
- Toner
- Serum: Incorporate a specialized serum, alternating with retinol.
- Face Mask: Treat your skin to a nourishing or clarifying mask.
- Moisturizer
- Eye Care

Weekly Treatments:

- Exfoliation: Use a gentle exfoliator 2-3 times a week.
- Face Mask: Apply a hydrating or detoxifying mask once a week.

Remember, consistency is key. Adjust based on your skin's response, and consult a skincare professional for personalized advice.

CONTENT

Acknowledgement...1

How to use this book 4

Bonus: 30-Day Skincare Routine............................7

CONTENT... 10

INTRODUCTION.. 10

CHAPTER 1: Understanding Aging.....................14

An Exemplified Explanation of the Science behind Aging 15

Common Signs and Symptoms of Aging 17

CHAPTER 2: Lifestyle Changes............................ 22

Importance of a balanced diet for anti-aging.......... 23

The role of hydration and its impact on skin health 30

Incorporating regular exercise into your routine..... 31

CHAPTER 3: Skincare Routine...............................34

Basics of a skincare routine for anti-aging..............36

Choosing the right products for your skin type....... 40

CHAPTER 4: Stress Management........................... 49

Exploring the link between stress and aging 50

Techniques for managing stress and promoting relaxation.. 52

CHAPTER 5: Quality Sleep.................................... 53

Understanding the importance of sleep in anti-aging. 54

CHAPTER 6: Mind-Body Connection 61

Exploring practices like meditation and mindfulness 63

CHAPTER 7: Supplements and Anti-Aging..............69

Overview of supplements that may support anti-aging...72

CHAPTER 8: Building Healthy Habits......................75

The importance of tracking and documenting your anti aging growth................................. 76

CONCLUSION...79

GLOSSARY...81

REVIEW PAGE...87

INTRODUCTION

Aging is a complicated and intriguing process that is an inescapable journey that signifies the passage of time on the canvas of our lives. Our bodies change throughout time in a variety of ways, some visible and some hidden beneath the surface. Anyone attempting to withstand the passage of time must comprehend the complex interactions between these processes.

The biochemical dance between our genes and environment is what drives aging. Our complex code, known as our DNA, is what controls our growth, development, and eventually aging processes. Our cells' once-efficient machinery eventually becomes less precise with age, which has a cascade of impacts that can take many different forms. On the outside, the first indications of aging are frequently seen on our skin, which is the body's outermost layer and a testament to the years that pass. While the skin loses part of its youthful flexibility, wrinkles tell stories of laughter and experience. These apparent alterations are caused by the slow loss of the proteins collagen and elastin, which give skin its structure and suppleness. The wider fight against aging is symbolized by the fight against fine lines. Internally, aging has an affect on almost every organ and function in the body, not just the skin. Once unwavering and unflappable, bones lose density and become increasingly brittle. Once flexible and strong, joints can become stiff and uncomfortable due to wear and strain. Changes in blood vessels and heart function can impact general vitality and the cardiovascular system, which is the beating heart of life.

Aging causes changes in the body's metabolism, which is the complex engine that turns fuel into energy. Weight management becomes a complex problem when the rate at which calories are burned starts to decrease. Decreases in muscle mass, which is important for strength and mobility, can lead to weariness and a weakened immune system.

The nervous system, which is our bodies' complex communication network, changes on its own. The messengers that carry messages, called neurons, often have difficulties continuing to operate at their best. The delicate changes that can occur in cognitive abilities, the symphony of memory and processing speed, underline the significance of mental health in the aging process.

The immune system, which is our body's first line of defense, may face challenges in its capacity to successfully fight off infections and illnesses throughout these changes. Hormones are chemical messengers that regulate a variety of biological activities. Their delicate balance can alter and affect mood, energy levels, and general vigor.

Understanding that aging is a unique experience is crucial to accepting the journey that comes with growing older. Every person has a distinct story that is shaped by a combination of environmental influences, lifestyle decisions, and genetics. While there are certain aspects of aging that we cannot control, we do have the ability to impact and maximize our well-being by the decisions we make.

The facts of how aging affects the body are not universal; rather, it is a tapestry influenced by factors such as environment, lifestyle, and heredity. There is a constant conversation going on between the years we have lived and the years to come. A comprehensive strategy for anti-aging that includes fostering vitality, resilience, and general well-being in addition to the quest for young aesthetics can be achieved by welcoming this journey with awareness and purpose.

Adopting anti-aging techniques is a significant investment in the quality of our lives, rather than a pursuit of perpetual youth. Adopting these habits becomes a pledge to a vibrant, healthy future and a statement of self-care as the years pass. By taking care of our bodies with a nutritious diet, consistent exercise, and a conscientious skincare regimen, we strengthen the resilience of our internal systems and resist the outward signs of aging.

Anti-aging techniques touch on the core of our wellbeing and go beyond appearances. They enable us to preserve our mental acuity, emotional equilibrium, and agility. These practices are essentially a realization that our bodies are temples that require conscious maintenance. Accepting anti-aging means setting out on a path of self-respect, with the light of our health illuminating our way.

CHAPTER 1:
Understanding Aging

The study of aging, or gerontology, is committed to comprehending and managing every element that contributes to a person's limited life. Debility is a major aspect of human experience, but it is not the only thing it addresses; a far wider variety of phenomena are covered. Each species has a life history in which the total life span is proportional to the reproductive life span, the technique of reproduction, and the developmental trajectory. Evolutionary biology and gerontology both benefit from understanding how these relationships came to be. It is imperative to differentiate between the solely physicochemical mechanisms of aging and the inadvertent organismic processes of illness and harm culminating in demise.

An Exemplified Explanation of the Science behind Aging

Aging is the gradual physiological alterations that cause an organism to age and eventually reach senescence, or a reduction in biological capacities and metabolic stress tolerance. Over time, aging can occur in a single cell, one organ, or the entire organism. It is a process that every adult living thing experiences throughout its lifetime. Aging refers to the gradual and systematic alterations in an organism that raise the likelihood of illness, mortality, and debility. Senescence is made up of several aging-related symptoms.

Think of your body as a large team, with small workers known as cells representing each member. Over time, these employees begin to relax and cease performing some jobs. For them, this is a normal aspect of life, akin to a break. Telomeres are one factor contributing to this split. Consider telomeres to be similar to the workers' headgear. These caps get smaller the more they labor. When the hats become too small, the employees determine it's time for a break and take a short break from work. Imagine your body right now as a busy factory. DNA is a set of instructions found inside every worker, or cell. These instructions are susceptible to slight alterations over time, just like mechanical wear and tear. The workers have a repair staff, but as time passes, they may not be as swift, which could result in some errors in the instructions. There are power plants called mitochondria in the factory's energy division. Similar to sparks from a machine, they generate some waste as they operate. These sparks may eventually inflict some harm.

The factory has some background noise, such as a humming sound. The way the workers respond to their surroundings is as follows. However, prolonged periods of this buzzing may lead to other issues, such as factory tool breakage. Regarding the protective hats (telomeres), telomerase is a little cofactor that can replenish some of the material in the caps. It's like giving them a little TLC so the laborers may continue for a while.

Epigenetics is another conductor in the workplace that tells the workers when to labor harder or slower. Over time, the conductor may alter the plan, which would have an impact on the factory's output.

Imagine now that you have some magical employees (stem cells) that can do a wide range of tasks. Over time, they may become less proficient in their roles, which could make it more difficult for the factory to make corrections.

Last but not least, hormones serve as messengers in the factory, directing everyone's actions. Over time, these messengers may modify their instructions, which could have an impact on the factory's operations.

Your body functions as a large team as a result. A bit like making sure the factory runs smoothly and everyone can enjoy a nice, long career, researchers are like detectives seeking to understand how this team works and create strategies to keep it running well for a long period of time.

Common Signs and Symptoms of Aging

By recognizing what changes are normal with age and what aren't, you may take little actions to try to slow down or even reverse the effects and have a better body.

Your heart pumps blood more forcefully: This is because, as you age, your arteries and blood vessels stiffen. Pumping blood requires more effort from your heart. Heart issues, including hypertension, may result from this one.

Help Tips: Continue being busy. You can lower your blood pressure and maintain a healthy weight by engaging in even a little daily exercise, such as swimming, running, or walking.

To maintain heart health, consume a diet high in fruits, vegetables, and whole grains. Take control of your stress. Make time for sleep. You may help rebuild and restore your heart and blood vessels by getting 7 to 8 hours of sleep every night.

It's possible that you've noticed a change in the texture and suppleness of your skin: The reason behind this is that, as you age, your skin produces less natural oil. In addition, there is a decrease in sweating and a partial loss of subcutaneous fat. It could appear thinner as a result. In addition, you might spot skin tags, wrinkles, age spots, and other small skin growths.

Help Tips: Bathe and shower in warm water; hot water dries the skin. Whenever you're outside, put on protective gear and sunscreen. If you see any changes to your skin, such as moles, check it frequently and report them to your doctor.

You have difficulties perceiving and hearing: You can have trouble concentrating on near objects. Perhaps this is the first time you'll require reading glasses. Maybe the light changes abruptly and you have trouble adjusting, or you perceive more glare. Your hearing may be impaired to the point that it becomes difficult for you to hear high frequencies or to follow discussions in a busy area.

Help Tips: Make routine check-ups for your hearing and eyesight. For eye protection outside, put on sunglasses. To avoid or filter loud noises, put on earplugs.

Loss of gums and teeth: It's possible that you'll detect a tug in your gums from your teeth. Your mouth may feel dry after taking some medications. Your risk of infections and tooth decay may increase if you have a dry mouth.

Help Tips: To get food and plaque out of the spaces between your teeth, brush twice a day and floss once. It offers the best defense against tooth loss and gum disease. Schedule routine cleanings and examinations at the dentist.

Increased Brittleness in Your Bones: Your bone density starts to decline as early as your 40s and 50s. Both their density and brittleness decrease. There might be some risk of fracture, due to this. Even if you appear shorter, you may still get their attention. Really, you may lose one to two inches of height starting in your 40s. The shrinking of your spine's disks causes it. It could feel more rigid in your joints. With aging comes a reduction in fluid and wear and tear on the cartilage lining joints. It's possible for you to get arthritis as the tissues separating your joints deteriorate.

Help Tips: Be careful to get adequate amounts of vitamin D and calcium. Dairy products, almonds, and veggies like kale and broccoli are good sources of calcium for you to consume. Supplements prescribed by your doctor may also be of help. Because it facilitates calcium absorption and maintains bone strength, vitamin D is essential for bone health. By spending time in the sun, some individuals are able to obtain adequate amounts of this vitamin. Sardines, egg yolks, tuna, and fortified foods, including milk and certain cereals, are further sources of it. Find out if you require a supplement from your doctor.

Using the restroom: Your bladder control may become more difficult. Roughly 10% of adults 65 and older experience it. A significant amount of urine is lost by some of these individuals before they can reach the restroom, while many of them just sneeze or cough occasionally. Menopause may play a role for women. Men's problems may stem from an enlarged prostate.

Not being as regular as you used to be may also be noticeable. Your bowel movement may become slower if you have diabetes, for example. Constipation can be caused by some medications. Blood pressure, seizures,

Parkinson's disease, and depression are among the conditions these drugs treat. Other causes of constipation include iron supplements and narcotic painkillers.

Help Tips: Consult with your doctor if you frequently feel the need to "go." Generally, it is possible to manage or even cure symptoms. Avoid alcohol, sodas, caffeine, and acidic meals as much as possible. These can worsen the situation.

In addition to helping with bladder control, Kegel exercises can tighten your pelvic floor muscles. Holding your poop, squeeze as hard as you can. Ten seconds of waiting, followed by five seconds of relaxation. Several times a day, repeat this four or five times in succession.

Eat lots of fruits, vegetables, and whole grains foods high in fiber to prevent constipation. Have a lot of water. Do your best to work out each day. It might facilitate defecation.

Muscle loss: finding my way around and maintaining my strength is harder. Muscle loss with aging can cause weakness and a decrease in activity.

Help Tips: Whether it's a quick stroll or light weightlifting, get some moderate exercise each day. Muscle tone and function will improve. To find the ideal amount of activity for you, consult your doctor. Consume a lot of vegetables, fruits, and lean meats like chicken and fish. Foods high in saturated fat and sugar should be avoided. also consume fewer servings. The number of calories you require is probably lower now than it was.

You also change in your sexual life: Women experience drier, thinner, and less elastic vaginal tissues during menopause. That could lessen the enjoyment of having sex. Smaller and less full-looking breasts can result from tissue and fat loss. Men may experience difficulty achieving or maintaining an erection as they get older.

Help Tips: See your physician. They may recommend drugs to reduce physical discomfort or increase your libido. There is no going back in time. We may, however, take optimal advantage of our bodies as we age by being patient, careful, and making wise lifestyle adjustments.

CHAPTER 2: Lifestyle Changes

This chapter serves as a traveling guide to help you stay vibrant and young. We are discussing daily matters such as proper skin care, diet, and exercise. Consider it a handbook filled with simple advice on how to incorporate these changes into your everyday life. You can maintain your energy and feel better with small adjustments rather than making drastic changes. Thus, let's integrate these anti-aging practices into your daily routine, whether it's eating healthily or exercising.

Importance of a balanced diet for anti-aging

Our qualities in life, fitness, looks, and risk of disease can all be significantly impacted by the foods we eat as we get older. The normal aging process in our bodies is supported by a variety of nutrients. By supporting healthy skin, for example, certain nutrients may help delay the aging process. It's crucial to remember that diet is just one facet of aging gracefully; eating certain meals won't help you seem significantly younger.

Even so, incorporating foods high in nutrients into your diet will help you feel and look your best as you age. Generally speaking, aim to eat:

- nutritious protein sources
- wholesome fats

- foods high in antioxidant content

These ten nutrient-dense foods promote healthy aging.

1. Olive oil, extra virgin

Among the healthiest oils available is extra virgin olive oil. It has a lot of antioxidants and good fats, which help the body fight inflammation and oxidative damage brought on by an imbalance of free radicals. A diet high in olive oil has been associated with a decreased risk of long-term illnesses such as:

- Heart disease
- Metabolic syndrome
- Type 2 diabetes
- Some cancer types

Most notably, monounsaturated fats (MUFAs) account for roughly 73% of the fat in olive oil. Due to the potent anti-inflammatory properties of these beneficial fats, some research has indicated that a diet high in MUFAs may help prevent the aging of the skin. Additionally, extra virgin olive oil is rich in phenolic compounds with anti-inflammatory qualities and antioxidants like beta carotene and tocopherols.

Indeed, a 2012 study discovered that patients with severe skin aging were less likely to eat a diet high in monounsaturated fatty acids (MUFAs) from olive oil. The effect was most likely caused by the antioxidants and MUFAs in olive oil, which have anti-inflammatory qualities, according to the scientists. Cold-pressed extra virgin olive oil is the best option because it is less processed and has more antioxidants than oils that are extracted through other techniques. Test it with a salad or a dip.

2. Herbal tea

Because of its high antioxidant content, green tea can aid the body's battle against free radicals. Free radicals are unstable molecules that are produced as a result of regular cell activity. They may also develop in reaction to environmental stresses like tobacco smoke or ultraviolet (UV) light. If your cells have a high concentration of free radicals, they might cause harm.

Antioxidants can help with it. In order to prevent free radicals from causing harm, these molecules stabilize them. Antioxidants are typically obtained from foods such as green tea. Antioxidants known as polyphenols are especially abundant in green tea. In particular, it contains a lot of gallic acid, catechins, and epigallocatechin gallate (EGCG).

These might lower your chance of:
- heart conditions
- neurological deterioration
- early aging and other long-term conditions

Green tea's polyphenols may prevent free radicals from damaging the skin, thereby reducing the signs of external aging caused by environmental stressors like pollution and sunlight. Because green tea extract has anti-aging and antioxidant qualities, it is actually a common ingredient in skin care products. But before green tea products are suggested to prevent skin aging, additional research is required. Nevertheless, a diet rich in antioxidants is linked to a lower chance of developing chronic illnesses and better skin. Additionally, a wonderful way to increase the amount of antioxidants in your diet is to consume green tea.

3. Fatty Fish Foods

Foods high in fat can help maintain healthy skin. One such item is fatty fish. Heart disease, inflammation, and numerous other problems can be prevented by its long-chain omega-3 fats. Additionally, studies have demonstrated that omega-3 fatty acids are associated with a robust skin barrier and may aid in reducing inflammation that harms the skin.

One of the most well-liked forms of fatty fish, salmon, contains other qualities that can improve the health of your skin. First, salmon's pink hue is attributed to astaxanthin, an antioxidant pigment found in it. In one study, participants with sun-damaged skin took astaxanthin and collagen supplements for a duration of 12 weeks. They consequently saw a noticeable increase in the suppleness and moisture of their skin. Though they look promising, it's unclear if the benefits were caused by collagen, astaxanthin, or both. Moreover, protein, which is necessary for your body to make collagen and elastin, is abundant in salmon and other fatty fish. The suppleness, strength, and plumpness of skin are all due to these two molecules. Consuming proteins aids in the healing of wounds.

Lastly, fish have a lot of selenium. In addition to its involvement in DNA synthesis and repair, this mineral and antioxidant may help lessen and perhaps prevent UV-induced skin damage. Enough levels in the body may lessen the severity of skin conditions such as psoriasis.

4. cocoa or dark chocolate

Polyphenols, which have antioxidant properties in the body, are abundant in dark chocolate.

In particular, it includes flavonols, which are associated with several health advantages, such as a lower risk of:

- cognitive impairment
- cardiac disease
- type 2 diabetes

Furthermore, consuming a diet high in flavonols and other antioxidants is believed to help shield the skin from UV rays and slow down the aging process of the skin.

When compared to the control group, participants in high-quality 24-week research who drank a cocoa beverage high in flavanols saw a significant improvement in their skin elasticity and face wrinkles.

These are encouraging results, but other research has not found any benefits of dark chocolate for aging or skin appearance.

Always keep in mind that flavanol content increases with cocoa content. Whichever dark chocolate you decide to include in your diet, be sure it has minimal added sugar and at least 70% cocoa solids.

8. Guacamoles

Avocados are a great source of fiber, heart-healthy fats, and many vital vitamins and minerals. Due to their strong antioxidant content, they may be able to combat free radicals that age and harm the skin, while their high monounsaturated fat content may support a healthy skin membrane. A diet high in plant-based fats, for instance, has been associated with improved skin health in older people, according to one study. Avocados are a tasty and versatile food that can easily be included in your diet to provide additional nourishment for good skin.

9. Lettuces

Due in part to their high lycopene content, tomatoes offer an astonishing array of health benefits. Tomatoes get their red color from a type of pigment called lycopene. Additionally, it serves as an antioxidant to lower the chance of developing chronic illnesses. Lycopene may also offer a tiny degree of protection against the sun's harmful rays, according to studies done on human skin samples. But compared to wearing sunscreen, this protection is far less effective.

According to one study, after 15 weeks of daily consumption of an antioxidant-rich beverage containing lycopene, soy isoflavones, fish oil, and vitamins C and E, women's wrinkle depth decreased noticeably. Since the beverage also included a number of other substances, the study was unable to establish a direct link between lycopene and these skin advantages. The body absorbs lycopene much more readily when tomatoes are paired with healthful fats like avocado or olive oil.

10. The peptides in collagen

The most common type of protein in the body is collagen. Specifically, the skin and joints contain large concentrations of it. Our bodies start to break down collagen as we get older and generate it less efficiently. This may result in the progressive appearance of wrinkles and sagging skin.

Eating foods that promote collagen production will help you maintain the health of your skin for longer, even though this process is unavoidable and a normal aspect of aging. Among them are foods high in protein and vitamin C. Additionally beneficial is avoiding behaviors that hasten the degradation of collagen. These practices include smoking cigarettes and sunbathing in the sun.

Hydrolyzed collagen peptides, a smaller form of collagen that your body absorbs far more rapidly, have also been demonstrated in human tests to improve skin elasticity, hydration, and firmness while minimizing wrinkles. That being said, a lot of research ignores additional lifestyle variables like smoking, total diet, and protein consumption. Collagen-derived protein is used by the body wherever it is required, so the skin may not always use it.

The bottom line seems to be that eating a diet high in protein is essential for having good skin. Concentrate on eating a diet high in protein, and if you'd like to increase your intake even more, take a collagen supplement. Regularly consume these nutritious foods high in protein:

- Fish, eggs, and chicken tofu

The things you put in your mouth might affect your skin's health, especially as it ages. Foods rich in protein, good fats, and antioxidants have been associated with the greatest skin benefits. In addition to maintaining an active lifestyle, using the right skin care products, avoiding smoking, applying sunscreen, and eating a diet rich in whole, plant-based foods, think about adopting other skin-protecting practices.

The role of hydration and its impact on skin health

It's critical for general health to consume enough water each day. Water facilitates the removal of toxins from the body and skin, as well as digestion, circulation, and absorption. Although it can't hurt, not everyone will concur that drinking more water can enhance skin. Increasing water intake is generally associated with glowing skin, according to numerous reports. Acne sufferers have experienced the same outcomes. The effects of prolonged water consumption on skin health were examined in detail in a 2007 study published in the International Journal of Cosmetic Science. According to the study, for four weeks, consuming 2.25 liters (9.5 cups) of water daily changed the thickness and density of the skin. Drinking 500 milliliters of water, or around two cups, enhanced blood flow to the skin, according to a second University of Missouri–Columbia study.

Skin seems duller, and pores and wrinkles are more noticeable when not drinking enough water. Enough water keeps the skin hydrated and makes it more elastic, which makes it less prone to crack, irritate, and have blemishes. In order to keep your skin hydrated, Dr. Deliduka advises being proactive in all aspects of your life. "To maintain the health of your skin, don't just drink water. For optimal results, maintain a balance between skin care products and water. Immediately following a shower, Dr. Deliduka advises using a moisturizing moisturizer. Dr. Deliduka stated, "After showering, the skin is still porous and vulnerable to products, allowing for better absorption." To keep your skin hydrated and functioning correctly, aim to consume at least 8 glasses of water each day. You should be able to observe the effects of increased water intake on your own skin within just a few weeks, though results won't materialize instantly.

Incorporating regular exercise into your routine

Now, let's explore the realm of exercise - not the kind that makes you feel like a prisoner, but rather a daily celebration of what your body is capable of. This chapter is all about getting up, moving, and living a life that makes you feel good, no matter how many candles are on your birthday cake.

The Enchantment of Motion: Your body's greatest ally and companion on the journey to elegant aging is exercise. It's a daily injection of vitality that everybody can enjoy; it's not just for gym rats or elite athletes. Consider it a magic bullet that increases your vitality, keeps your heart pumping, and is the main character in the anti-aging story.

Discovering Your Sound: There is no one-size-fits-all approach to exercise. It's all about figuring out what works for you, much like when you meet your ideal dancing partner. Enjoying the exercise, regardless of the form it takes—a leisurely yoga flow, a lively dance class in your living room, or a quick stroll—is essential. This is your energetic, personal dance, and you are the choreographer.

The Game of Consistency: Have you ever heard the adage, "It's not what happens once in a while, but what happens every day that counts"? That certainly holds true in this case. The key to transforming exercise from an irregular occurrence into a daily routine is consistency. It's about showing up and allowing the exercise to become as natural as brushing your teeth, not about setting records. Instances of Activities to Adopt:

1. **Walking**: is a timeless exercise. Put on your sneakers and go for a walk in your community or a neighboring park. It's a terrific technique to declutter your mind and is gentle and effective.

2. **Dancing**: Create a dance floor in your living room. Let loose and enjoy yourself, whether it's with your favorite music or a dancing fitness DVD. It's about sensing the beat, not about being flawless.

3. **Yoga: is a** lovely blend of movement and awareness. Strength, flexibility, and calmness are all provided by yoga. You only need to discover a flow that works for you; you don't have to be a human pretzel.

4. Traversing: Riding a bike, whether stationary or in a park, is a low-impact workout that increases heart rate and leg movement.

5. Swimming: This workout is great for joints and is refreshing. Swimming exercises the entire body and utilizes many muscle groups. Plus, being in the water has a calming effect.

6. Strength Training: Don't let the weights scare you. Including strength training helps maintain muscular mass, which tends to decrease with age, even with little dumbbells or resistance bands.

7. Pilates: is an excellent exercise to improve your core. Pilates can help with posture, flexibility, and stability since it emphasizes regulated movements.

8. Backpacking: Hiking is an excellent way to get exercise and appreciate nature if you enjoy being outside. It's a moderately intense exercise that stimulates your body and mind.

Including Exercise in Your Daily Routine

Make everything flow smoothly. Perhaps it's choosing to use the stairs rather than the elevator, stretching briefly during your work break, or throwing a little dance party while preparing supper. Consistent little efforts pay out handsomely.

Cognitive Motion

Exercise is a mindful discipline as well as a physical activity. Enjoy the feeling of movement, pay attention to how your body feels, and use it as a way to take care of yourself. It's about accepting progress rather than striving for perfection.

The Advantages Against Aging

Frequent exercise is like giving your body a magical potion. It releases feel-good endorphins and improves joint health and circulation. Your muscles maintain their peak condition, and your heart becomes a happier organ. Additionally, exercise improves balance, coordination, and flexibility, all important components of the beautiful dance of aging.

Including regular exercise in your schedule will make you feel great as well as look great. It's about building a physique that will be your lifelong friend, having the stamina to enjoy life's small joys, and being resilient in the face of adversity. Now put on your sneakers, turn up the music, and start dancing energetically.

CHAPTER 3: Skincare Routine

A simple skin care regimen maintains your skin healthy and clean, yet it requires fewer steps than an elaborate one. The steps can change based on how much time you have and what you require. A standard regimen often entails removing makeup, washing your face, treating any imperfections on the spot, using sunscreen during the day, and applying moisturizer.

Don't feel compelled to complete every step in the lists above; not everyone enjoys a 10-step process.

Applying items from thinnest to thickest as you proceed through your skin care routine is, for the majority of people, a good rule of thumb, regardless of how many products you may be using. Finding a skin care regimen that suits you and that you will stick to is crucial. Enjoy playing around with it, whether it's a complex ceremony or something simpler. Beginning a skin care regimen is never too early or too late. By cleaning their faces when they wake up and before bed, as well as using sunscreen during the day, even children may learn the importance of skin care.

However, tailor your routine's stages and particular products to your age and skin conditions. Teenagers, for instance, could require a regimen centered around items to assist with the management of imperfections and oily skin. As they get older, adults could become increasingly interested in skincare products. Establish a regimen that works for you.

Basics of a skincare routine for anti-aging.

It's never too early to begin treating certain issues (such as pigmentation, small wrinkles around the eyes, and dulling skin). If all you do for anti-aging is use a cleanser and sunscreen, that will work just as well; it doesn't have to be particularly elaborate.

Morning and Night Steps

1. Use cleaner both night and morning:
It's not enough to just wash your face once. Engelman says, "Double-cleanse," adding, "Stick with a gentle cleanser that will not strip your skin of natural oils and leave you more dehydrated than before."
Apply an oil-based product first, then work up a lather with a gel-based cleanser to

ensure a proper double-clean. The debris, oil, and balm will dissolve the old makeup, and the gel follow-up guarantees a clean canvas for unobstructed pores and improved product absorption.

2. Toner in the Morning and Night

Toner follows the cleanser. "Toner is a necessary step for those who tend to have skin that is on the oily side, or if you are acne-prone," says Henry to me. Biologique's exfoliates and tones the skin with salicylic acid and phenol; Engelman suggests trying something similar. In addition to preparing your skin for the remainder of your regimen, this helps preserve the ideal pH balance of your skin.

Morning Steps

1. Vitamin C Serum (Morning Step):

What comes next? The serum. Vitamin C is the finest, according to Darden. "Vitamin C is an antioxidant that protects your skin from sun damage and free radicals,"

This velvety-smooth serum, enriched with 15% THD ascorbate (vitamin C), is intended to help balance and brighten your complexion. It also helps to improve the texture of your skin when combined with glycolic acid.

2. Apply face oil (morning step):

Apply a drop of this face oil to your extremely dry skin before putting on your daily moisturizer. It promises to keep your skin hydrated throughout the day and aid in the restoration of firmness and suppleness.

Rich in skin-beneficial components, including conditioning sea buckthorn oil and calming rosehip, this hydrating oil looks stunning on your vanity.

Rub a drop between your palms and gently press it into your face to avoid that oily sheen.

3. Moisturizer (morning step):
Allow it to absorb for a moment after applying your oil. Next, use a moisturizing product. Because of its fluffy texture and short ingredient list, our crew likes this Allies of Skin choice. This moisturizer, which is specifically made to aid with age issues, is bursting with probiotics and antioxidants. The texture is incredible—smooth, silky, and quite light—in addition to being effective.

4. SPF (morning steps):

The most crucial element of an anti-aging skincare regimen is SPF because the sun is a primary cause of premature aging. Its smooth texture is enhanced by the presence of hyaluronic acid, which gives the skin moisture and plumpness. If you're worried about chemical sunscreens, check for options free of oxybenzone.

Weekly and at Night Steps

1. Apply a face mask (weekly and at night):

Making face masks is a nice way to spend a quiet evening, but it's also a terrific way to use them in the morning after doing your double cleaning.

"The purpose of masks is to strengthen and hydrate the skin barrier," says Darden. "Full of peptides, ceramides, and hyaluronic acid, they support collagen production, which can smooth lines and wrinkles."

2. Retinol (weekly and at night):

Retinol is the most crucial component of an anti-aging regimen, according to Darden, aside from sunscreen. "Retinol effectively reduces the appearance of fine lines and helps stop new wrinkles from developing. Additionally, because of cellular turnover, it will aid in reducing pigmentation," she says.

To see a noticeable improvement in the texture and color of your skin, apply this face oil before moisturizing. It's made especially to encourage the formation of collagen and elastin. Avocado seed oil plumps up skin, while blue tansy and German chamomile reduce redness.

3. Serum (weekly and at night):

Engelman suggests using serum AHAs, like glycolic acid, for exfoliation. This alternative with lactic acid brightens and moisturizes the skin. Prickly pear extract calms skin, and lemongrass and licorice lighten dark areas. Every few nights, use it under your moisturizer and on top of my Luna sleeping oil.

4. Moisturizer (weekly and at night):

According to Engelman, peptides and ceramides are essential ingredients because they "reinforce the integrity of the skin." It feels as light as a green smoothie applied to your skin. This is the moisturizer to use if you want to target aging concerns because it is packed with nutrients and active components, specifically pygmy water lily stem cell extract and soybean folic acid, which are created to induce greater collagen creation.

5. Eye Care (weekly and at night):

Since the skin around our eyes is "thinner than the rest of the face and therefore needs a little extra attention," Engelman reminds us that eye cream is a necessity. Hydrating the area beneath your eyes is crucial since it keeps the skin firm and supple and minimizes the appearance of wrinkles! A hyaluronic acid serum can be applied before your moisturizer if you feel that you need more moisture.

Choosing the right products for your skin type

Beautiful skin is characterized by its rich, even hue, vivid glow, and silky-smooth texture. If that's your goal, you need to create a strong skincare regimen that includes selecting the appropriate products. Although initially daunting, with a little understanding, you'll find yourself navigating the skincare industry like an expert. The selection of skincare products, which range from high-end creams and serums to masks and ointments, can be intimidating, particularly if you don't know what you're looking for or where to start. Because every person's skin type is different, understanding how to create a customized skincare routine with the proper products will help you achieve your skincare objectives.

For dry skin: look for products with lactic acid and shea butter. "These ingredients provide hydration and mild exfoliation to keep dry skin looking radiant," according to Dr. Green.

For sensitive skin: Seek out items with aloe vera, oats, and shea butter if you have sensitive skin. "They hydrate well and don't usually cause breakouts in people."

To begin, use these pointers:

1. Identify the type of skin you have: When it comes to creating a skincare routine, the best place to start is by getting to know your skin type. Determine whether you have oily, dry, sensitive, or mixed skin. The idea is to supplement your program with items made specifically for your type of skin.

Suppose that despite having dry skin, you select a product designed for oily skin. Your skin is already dry; you'll exacerbate it. Do your research beforehand since without understanding what type of skin you have, it is impossible to select the appropriate products.

2. Be Aware of your needs: Consider your skin's requirements for a while. Maybe you wish to blur some small lines on your body. Perhaps you wish to reduce the look of wide pores or persistent acne that isn't improving with your usual regimen. The goods you select must adequately address the problems that most worry you.

3. Recognize theFundamentals: The four skincare commandments are the cornerstone of any effective program, regardless of your skin type. Observe these commandments:

- **Cleanse:** Regardless of your skin type, you ought to use a gentle cleanser that doesn't dry out your complexion. Even though you might not realize it, your skin picks up bacteria, grime, and other impurities all day long. Your skin feels refreshed after using a decent cleanser, which gets rid of dead skin cells, excess oil, and other contaminants.

- **Hydrate:** In addition to seeming more radiant, plump, and healthy, well-hydrated skin is also more resistant to problems like wrinkles. For this reason, any skincare routine should include a good moisturizer. Your epidermis and dermis need a constant flow of water. Hyaluronic acid is one of the important chemicals to look for in hydrating cosmetics since it draws and holds moisture in the skin.

- **Defend:** Mother nature can wreak havoc on your skin with everything from UV damage to excessive humidity. Weather can harm your skin and hasten the aging process, in addition to making it look lifeless and drab. It can also aggravate skin sensitivity. A product to shield your skin from the elements of everyday life is essential to any skincare routine.

Resilient components such as antioxidants and vital fatty acids contribute to the continuous radiance of your skin. It's imperative that the broad-spectrum SPF be at least 30.

- **Treat:** A daily go-to treatment for the most serious problems with your skin is essential. Investing in the everyday health of your skin is money well spent, whether your goal is anti-aging or discoloration fading. The substances you should avoid using depend on the main issues with your skin. For example, select products with anti-aging superstars like alpha hydroxy acids if wrinkles are an issue. These substances help your skin look more youthful by reducing fine wrinkles.

- **Consult a dermatologist:** A medical professional with expertise in all things skin care can help you make the best skincare product choices. If you're serious about maintaining good skin, visit a certified dermatologist as soon as possible. Dermatologists are knowledgeable about products and can offer advice to help you start off on the correct track, in addition to having a thorough understanding of your skin.

4. Refrain from believing the hype:

"Packaging and popularity are sometimes easy traps and shouldn't hold too much weight or value into what we select for our skin," explains Dr. David. If you're going to purchase a product on the advice of a friend or influencer, consider the type of skin that person was struggling with rather than just how nice their skin looks now. This will provide you with a more accurate sense of how well the product will function for you.

5. Look for these components:

Glycerin: Dr. David refers to glycerin as the foundational component of moisturizing products. Hyaluronic acid and ceramides are two significant, naturally occurring skin-moisturizing factors. Dr. David states that she looks for glycerins and ceramides in lotions and creams and prefers hyaluronic acid in serum form.

L-ascorbic acid (Vitamin C): Vitamin C, in particular the form of l-ascorbic acid, is an antioxidant that acts to counteract UV radiation damage and promote the formation of collagen.

Tocopherol, or vitamin E: Vitamin E and vitamin C are a potent skincare combination since they have qualities in common. Augustinus Bader's The Hand Treatment, which blends vitamin E with glycerin and shea butter, is a luxurious hand lotion that is worth spending a little extra on.

Retinol: An essential component to look for in products for your evening regimen is retinoid. Collagen is stimulated and skin cells are turned over. Vitamin B3, or niacinamide, is an excellent oil-controlling, skin-hydrating, and skin-tone-evening substance.

6. Steer clear of these ingredients.

Fragrance/parfum: It's crucial to stay away from added fragrances if you have sensitive skin since they might irritate and trigger skin allergies.

Sulfates: Sulfates are washing ingredients that are frequently present in shampoos and body washes. They might irritate skin and hair by removing their natural oils.

Parabens: As a chemical preservative that stops bacteria from growing, parabens are frequently added to items. They are recognized as what Dr. David and other industry professionals refer to as estrogen mimickers, and over time, their ability to upset hormonal equilibrium may be detrimental. Breast cancer patients and small children may find this challenging, as both Drs. David and Green warn.

Formaldehyde and its releasers: Since formaldehyde is regarded as a recognized carcinogen, it is uncommon to find it in an ingredient list these days. However, as Dr. David says, it's frequently swapped out with substances with alternative names (quaternium-15, imidazolidinyl urea, DMDM hydantoin, and so on) that gradually release formaldehyde to serve as a preservative. Although the safety of these components in this capacity has not been established, according to Dr. David, it is nevertheless advisable to be on the lookout for any potential allergies.

7. Be aware that better doesn't necessarily equate to natural: While seeing familiar terms in the ingredients list can be reassuring, it doesn't always mean that's the safest option. Sometimes reading the terms "natural" and "organic" on a product label is just a marketing ploy. Furthermore, a product may occasionally be designated as natural even when it only contains one or two of the listed constituents.

8. Observe the ingredient order: After you've determined the main ingredients to target or stay away from, you should focus on where those substances are located on the ingredients list. Dr. David suggests, as a general guideline, focusing on the first five ingredients as they often make up around 80% of the contents of the product.

The ingredients in the product will be listed from highest to lowest concentration, so if any of the first five ingredients are known to cause issues or irritation, you should avoid that product.

9. Be at ease with the lengthy component list:

We're frequently trained to seek foods with shorter, more recognizable ingredient lists when choosing what to put in our bodies. When it comes to getting the most out of your skincare products, a shorter list could be simpler to understand, but it might not always meet your needs.

Naturally, the components list will get a little lengthier if you're looking for anti-aging qualities or planning to purchase skincare items made to a medical grade.

10. Make use of your abilities: Choosing skincare products with the proper ingredients doesn't require you to be a walking dictionary. Utilize internet resources to make things easier. For ingredient and product research, Dr. David recommends using two online databases.

11. Perform a patch test every time: Using a patch test is a wise move when it comes to your product removal process. Furthermore, it's a fantastic justification to visit Ulta or Sephora without breaking the bank.

To find out if specific substances or products can irritate your skin, clog your pores, or trigger allergic responses, you can perform a patch test. "I believe the key takeaway is to cease using the product if it's aggravating your skin or making it worse; it's not the correct one for you.

Importance of sunscreen

At any age, one of the greatest and simplest ways to safeguard the health and beauty of your skin is to wear sunscreen. Regular use of sunscreen guards against sunburn, skin cancer, and premature aging.

What is SPF protection?

The effectiveness of a sunscreen to shield against UVB radiation, a particular type of ultraviolet light, is indicated by the sun protection factor (SPF). Skin cancer and sunburns are caused by UVB radiation. There are two other forms of ultraviolet light: UVA rays (which cause skin aging and cancer) and UVC rays (which do not penetrate the earth's atmosphere). UVB and UVA radiation can be warded off with a broad spectrum sunscreen.

Which brand of sunscreen is required for purchase?

Select a sunscreen with at least 30 SPF for daily use. Use a sunscreen with an SPF of at least 60 if you spend a lot of time outside. Because most people don't apply as much sunscreen as they should, this higher SPF helps make up for the fact that less sunscreen is actually applied. For everyone to manufacture vitamin D (which aids in the absorption of calcium for stronger and healthier bones), sun exposure is necessary. However, skin, eyes, and the immune system can all suffer harm from unprotected exposure to the sun's ultraviolet (UV) radiation.

How much sunscreen is necessary?

You'll need around one ounce of sunscreen to protect your arms, legs, neck, and face. One ounce of sunscreen, squeezed into your hand, is sufficient to cover your palm entirely. About a half teaspoon will do to protect your face and neck.

Is sunscreen best applied last or should it come first?

Applying your skin care products in any order is irrelevant as long as the sunscreen is broad-spectrum, water-resistant, and has at least SPF 30. Working with bare skin—that is, without makeup or moisturizer—seems most comfortable to some people. Determine what your regimen requires. Consult your dermatologist if you are unsure about layering any particular products.

Does SPF-containing cosmetics work?

Even high-sPF makeup is insufficient to keep your skin safe. To achieve the indicated SPF, you would need a lot more makeup than you usually apply.

Are sunscreens made of minerals that are superior?

Sunscreens are frequently divided into two types: mineral and chemical. Avobenzone, homosalate, octisalate, octocrylene, and other substances are used in chemical sunscreens. Titanium dioxide or zinc oxide are the ingredients in mineral sunscreens. Sunscreens made of chemicals and minerals function similarly in that they absorb UV light and convert it to very little heat. Additionally, mineral sunscreens reflect a tiny bit of UV radiation. Sunscreens with chemicals can sting certain people. Mineral sunscreen might be a better option if your skin is sensitive or if you react to cosmetics often. Mineral sunscreens have the drawback of frequently leaving a prominent white cast, especially on skin with pigment. Ot

Otherwise, that's a matter of preference. You should always opt for the best sunblock.

Is it truly necessary for me to reapply sunscreen during the day?

In general, reapplying sunscreen is advised every two hours, particularly after perspiring or swimming. A second application might not be necessary if you work indoors and keep your desk away from windows. But be careful how often you go outside. Simply for peace of mind, have an extra bottle of sunscreen on your desk. Your skin could be in danger even after a quick walk during lunch. Remember that there isn't a flawless sunscreen. When you can, find shade and put on sunglasses, wide-brimmed hats, or other protective gear.

CHAPTER 4: Stress Management

You can live a more balanced and healthier life by practicing stress management. Stress management provides numerous strategies for managing stress difficulties. An automatic bodily, mental, and emotional reaction to a challenging situation is stress. It is an everyday occurrence for all people. Positively, stress can spur development, activity, and transformation. Negative, persistent stress, however, can lower life quality.

Exploring the link between stress and aging

Unfortunately, stress is a necessary part of life, no matter what stage you're in. Aging is a normal aspect of life, much like stress. We might not experience as much physical or mental damage from stressful situations while we're young and strong. It becomes increasingly challenging to manage stress and anxiety as we age, though, as the body's natural defenses steadily weaken.

It may be argued that growing older itself can be stressful at times: adjusting to the death of a loved one, planning for future health and independence losses, and experiencing prolonged unemployment can all be quite confusing.

Thankfully, you (or your senior loved one) may manage your stress levels and make the most of senior living in a number of ways. Continue reading to find out more about how stress affects aging and discover stress management techniques for a gentle retirement.

What repercussions does stress have on the body?

Our bodies release stress hormones like cortisol and adrenaline when we're physically or emotionally upset. In order to properly handle the stressful circumstances at hand, these stress hormones can be useful in giving us short-term energy and focus. But over time, prolonged periods of stress can cause an excess of stress hormones, which can cause dangerous bodily imbalances. High blood pressure, heart disease, impaired immune systems, and memory loss have all been related to excess stress hormones. Furthermore, blood vessels may constrict and cause loss of vision and hearing when adrenaline is released continuously.

The brain's capacity to control stress hormone levels deteriorates with age. This causes older people to experience higher amounts of stress in addition to contributing to hormone abnormalities. Chronic stress makes it more likely for a person to make bad lifestyle choices, which exacerbates already existing health issues. Put another way, stress exacerbates aging, and aging exacerbates stress—a vicious cycle.

The body's cells are impacted by stress as well.Telomeres are the protective "caps" at the end of DNA chromosomes that are inevitably going to break down. Nonetheless, scientists have discovered that when the body is under stress, the process might quicken. The cells lose their protection when their telomeres are too short. Parkinson's disease, diabetes, cardiovascular disease, and cancer have all been related to shortened telomeres.

Techniques for managing stress and promoting relaxation

The good news is that managing your stress can help you feel better physically, and vice versa. Stress levels can drop when your health improves.

- Keep in touch with your loved ones. A positive social life can improve one's general health, quality of life, and sense of self. Actually, a number of disorders pertaining to both physical and mental health are associated with loneliness and isolation.

- Continue to be active. A little yoga practice or brisk 30-minute stroll might help elevate your attitude.

- Engage in mentally challenging activities to keep your mind bright, such as games, puzzles, and novels, with loved ones.

- Make sure you sleep well and in abundance.

- To improve both your physical and mental health, eat a well-balanced diet.

- Stay away from circumstances that are too stressful.

When it comes to managing chronic stress, some people might also benefit from using prescription drugs or professional mental health assistance. For more advice on how to enhance your health, it never hurts to speak with your physician or a mental health specialist.

CHAPTER 5: Quality Sleep

Modern life moves so quickly that there are moments when you can't even pause to relax. It may seem unreal to consistently enjoy a restful night's sleep. But sleep is just as vital to overall health as exercise and a balanced diet. Numerous illnesses and disorders are more likely to develop in those who don't routinely get enough good sleep. These include dementia and obesity, in addition to heart disease and stroke.

Understanding the importance of sleep in anti-aging

A good night's sleep is a powerful anti-aging tool that is essential to preserving general health and wellbeing. Not only does it feel good to be rested, but it's also an important part of the complex dance of slowing down the aging process. The following explains why sleep is a real anti-aging defender:

1. **Repair and regeneration of cells:** The body performs cellular regeneration and repair while you are in deep sleep. This results in a more youthful appearance through the regeneration of muscular tissues, skin cells, and other essential elements.

2. Endocrine System: Growth hormone is released when we sleep, and it is necessary for muscle growth, cell repair, and general renewal. Hormone balance is necessary to keep one's appearance fresh and young.

3. Collagen Production: Sleep is when the protein responsible for skin suppleness, collagen, is created. Insufficient sleep can result in a reduction in collagen production, which in turn can cause fine lines and wrinkles to appear.

4. Cognitive Ability and Memory: Getting enough sleep improves one's ability to think clearly, consolidate memories, and solve problems. Retaining a youthful mindset requires keeping your mind active.

5. Detoxification: Stress hormones can be controlled with adequate sleep. Good sleep functions as a natural stress reliever, encouraging a more calm and balanced state. Prolonged stress hastens the aging process.

6. Management of Inflammation: The regulation of inflammation in the body is influenced by sleep. Good sleep serves as a preventive measure against chronic inflammation, which is connected to a number of age-related illnesses.

7. System Support for Immunity: A well-rested body can fight off ailments more effectively. Restorative sleep strengthens the immune system and helps avoid the wear and tear that comes with recurrent diseases.

8. State of Mind and Emotional Health: Anger and mood fluctuations are frequently caused by sleep deprivation. Resilience on an emotional level is enhanced by getting enough sleep, which also improves mood and lessens the psychological effects of stress.

Essentially, getting enough sleep is like hitting the reset button for your body and mind. It provides a comprehensive method for preserving youth from the inside out, making it a cornerstone of anti-aging techniques. A healthy, more energetic, and graceful aging you can achieve by making sleep a priority. It's not only a luxury.

Tips for improving sleep quality

You could struggle to obtain enough good sleep every night, even though it's crucial for both physical and mental health. Your life is affected in every way by inadequate sleep. Your daily sleeping routine, sometimes referred to as "sleep hygiene," might improve your quality of sleep.

1. Make an Upgraded Bedding and Mattress Purchase: It is essential to make sure you are comfortable enough to unwind if you have the ideal mattress for your requirements and tastes. To prevent aches and pains in your spine, it is advisable to choose a supportive mattress and pillow. A big part of creating a cozy feeling in your bed is your bedding. Select bedding that is cozy to the touch and will aid in regulating body temperature while you sleep.

2. Turn off the lights: Your sleep and circadian cycle may be disrupted by excessive light exposure. Using a sleep mask over your eyes or blackout drapes over your windows can filter light and keep it from interfering with your sleep. Steering clear of strong light can aid in the shift from day to night and support your body's melatonin production, which induces sleep.

3. Reduce Noisiness: One of the most crucial aspects of creating a bedroom that promotes sleep is minimizing noise. Consider using a fan or white noise machine to drown out any adjacent noise sources if you are unable to remove them. Another way to block out noises while you try to fall asleep is to use headphones or earplugs.

4. Enter 65 to 68 degrees Fahrenheit on the thermostat: You don't want to be distracted by your bedroom's temperature by being overly hot or cold. While everyone has a different optimal temperature, the majority of research suggests sleeping in a room that is somewhat colder, between 65 and 68 degrees.

5. Sleep for a Minimum of Seven Hours: You must factor that time into your routine if you want to ensure that you obtain the appropriate amount of sleep each night. Determine a target bedtime that permits a minimum of seven hours of sleep by working backward from your fixed wake-up time. Give yourself extra time before bed to be ready for sleep whenever possible.

6. Set your daily alarm clock to the same time: If you are waking up at different times every day, it is very impossible for your body to adjust to a healthy sleep schedule.

Even on the weekends and other days when you might be tempted to sleep in, set a wake-up time and stick to it.

7. Try to limit naps to 20 minutes: Napping should be done carefully if you want to sleep through the night. Overly extended naps taken too late in the day can disrupt your sleep pattern and make it more difficult to fall asleep when you want to. Early afternoon, right after lunch, is the ideal time to take a sleep; a 20-minute nap is ideal.

8. Unwind for half an hour prior to going to sleep: Being comfortable makes it much simpler to go to sleep. To help you relax and prepare for sleep, try reading quietly, doing low-impact stretching, listening to relaxing music, and other relaxation techniques. Rather than trying to fall asleep, concentrate on attempting to relax. Progressive muscle relaxation, guided visualization, mindfulness meditation, and controlled breathing are a few relaxation techniques that can help you go asleep.

9. Turn Off Electronics One Hour Before Sleep: It can be difficult to fully unwind when using tablets, cellphones, and laptops because they keep your brain wired. Your body's natural melatonin production may also be suppressed by the light from these electronics. Prior to going to bed, make every effort to unplug for at least one hour.

10. Take in 30 Minutes of Natural Light: Light exposure controls the body's internal clock. Due to the powerful effects of sunlight, make an effort to step outside or let natural light in through open windows or blinds. Your circadian rhythm can be restored by exposing yourself to natural light early in the day. Speak with your doctor about utilizing a light therapy box if you are unable to use natural light.

11. Get 20 minutes or more of exercise every day: Frequent exercise has been shown to yield numerous health benefits, including the promotion of sound sleep through changes in body temperature and energy utilization. The majority of specialists recommend against engaging in strenuous exercise right before bed because it may make it more difficult for your body to fall asleep.

12. Avoid Using Coffee After 2:00 P.M.: Among the most consumed beverages worldwide are those that contain caffeine, such as sodas, tea, and coffee. Some people may find it tempting to try to fight daytime sleepiness with the energy boost that caffeine provides, but this strategy is unsustainable and may result in long-term sleep loss. Watch how much caffeine you consume and limit it later in the day when it can interfere with falling asleep.

13. Consider Your Drinking in the Hour Before Bed: Some people love having a nightcap before going to bed since alcohol can make you sleepy. It is advisable to abstain from alcohol in the hours before bed because it has negative effects on the brain that might impair the quality of sleep.

14. A few hours before going to bed, eat dinner: If your body is still processing a large dinner, it may be more difficult to fall asleep. Try to avoid late dinners and reduce your intake of particularly fatty or spicy foods to reduce the number of food-related sleep interruptions. Choose something light for your evening snack if you're hungry.

15. Minimize Smoke and Nicotine Exposure: A variety of sleep-related issues, such as trouble falling asleep and disrupted sleep, have been linked to smoke exposure, including secondhand smoke. As a stimulant, nicotine has been shown to interfere with sleep, especially when used in the evening.

16. Save your bed just for sex and sleep: It can be tempting to spend your free time in bed if your bed is comfy, but this can lead to issues when it is time to go to sleep. Make sure that the only things you do in bed are sleep and sex if you want to create a strong mental association between your bed and sleep.

17. Leave Your Bed After Twenty Minutes: It's important to prevent associating your bed with insomnia-related annoyance. Consequently, it is recommended to get out of bed and engage in a soothing activity in low light if you have been in bed for around 20 minutes and are still unable to fall asleep. Once you're exhausted, go back to bed and refrain from using electronics or checking the time.

18. Maintain a Sleep Diary: Keeping a sleep diary on a daily basis will help you monitor your sleep quality and pinpoint any situations that may be promoting or hindering your sleep. Your sleep diary can help you track the effectiveness of any new sleep schedule or other changes you are making to your sleep hygiene.

19. Examine add-ons: You might want to talk to your doctor about taking vitamins in addition to practicing better sleep hygiene generally. It's normal practice to use melatonin pills to reduce the amount of time it takes to fall asleep. Glycine, chamomile, and valerian are further natural sleep aids. The U.S. Food and Drug Administration does not strictly monitor dietary supplements, so it is crucial to take precautions to be sure you are buying reliable sleep aids.

20. Speak with a Physician: If you are having significant trouble falling asleep, your doctor is the best person to provide specific, tailored advice. If your sleep issues are getting worse, lingering longer than expected, posing a risk to your health or safety, or coexisting with other unexplained health issues, see your doctor. They can treat any underlying issues and offer more information.

CHAPTER 6: Mind-Body Connection

The interdependent relationship between mental and physical wellness is captured by the notion of the "mind-body connection." The idea that our attitudes, ideas, and behaviors can have a significant impact on our physical health and well-being is symbolized by this phrase. On the other hand, mental and emotional moods can be influenced by physical health just as much. It draws attention to the subtle ways that mental and emotional emotions can influence symptomatology, or bodily responses.

The interaction between the mental, emotional, and physical facets of health is characterized by the mind-body connection. Essentially, it pertains to our knowledge and comprehension of the connection between our mental and emotional well-being and our physical health. The essential idea of this relationship is that physical health can have an impact on mental and emotional states, and vice versa. Mental and emotional experiences can directly influence physical health.

The idea of a mind-body link has its roots in traditional therapeutic practices dating back to antiquity. "Holistic health," a paradigm that recognizes the interdependence of mind, body, and soul in reaching optimal health, was singled out by the ancient Greeks. The importance of emotional equilibrium for physical health was also emphasized by traditional Chinese medicine. But the medical establishment took a dualistic stance for most of the 20th century, treating the body and mind as distinct entities. The holistic approach to health theories of mind-body oneness has only been reexamined by health experts in the last few decades.

Exploring practices like meditation and mindfulness

In a nutshell, meditation is the discipline of calming the mind and paying attention to the breath. It's not as simple as it seems, particularly in the incredibly linked society of today. It requires a great deal of patience, openness, and practice. There are various forms of meditation; the following are the most widely used ones:

- **Being mindful Practice meditation:** focuses on being aware of the noises and goings-on around you at any given moment. You allow your thoughts to be aware of the noises without getting overly preoccupied. You can either walk or sit still while doing this.

- **Mantra (transcendental) Meditation:** During mantra meditation, one chants aloud certain syllables. The mantra "Om" is frequently employed in yoga, as you may already be aware, because it sends forth a deep vibration that facilitates concentration.

- **Spiritual Meditation:** In spiritual meditation, one can converse with a higher power through prayer, for example. It usually centers on a query or issue you may be experiencing.

- **Focused Meditation:** As the name suggests, this style of meditation concentrates on a mantra, sound, object, or idea. When you concentrate on anything, the million other thoughts that are racing through your mind start to fade.

The Advantages of Meditation for Anti-Aging

Anecdotally and scientifically, meditation has been shown to decrease stress, enhance focus, heighten self-awareness, strengthen the immune system, improve cardiovascular health, and slow down the aging process, to name a few advantages. These studies demonstrate the significance and magnitude of the benefits of meditation, even though it shouldn't be your primary anti-aging practice.

Meditation promotes healthy brain cells by reducing brain activity: Another significant change that occurs in our brains during meditation is a reduction in the amount of information that is processed, as demonstrated by magnetic resonance imaging (MRI) research. Researchers led by Harvard neurologist Dr. Sarah Lazar have shown that those who meditate have more gray matter, or brain cells, in their brains. This finding may explain why people who meditate have higher levels of compassion, reduced blood pressure, and improved memory, among other benefits.

Stress is reduced by meditation: Numerous scholars have expounded upon the significance of psychological or emotional stress in either precipitating or intensifying the aging processes. According to several prominent theories of aging, oxidative stress is the main cause of aging. Numerous studies have demonstrated decreased oxidative stress during meditation, as indicated by lower concentrations of malondialdehyde, lipid peroxides, and vanillylmandelic acid in the urine. It has been suggested that the decrease in these oxidative stress levels is due to our natural ability to repair and regenerate ourselves, which slows down the aging process.

Telomerase activity is elevated during meditation: The telomeres at the end of our chromosomes shorten with age, which is what causes us to age and eventually die. Enzymes called telomerase, which stop telomeres from shortening, are known to decline with age and are therefore a good indicator of long-term health. According to studies, having more stem cells and telomerase activity in our blood may improve our quality of life and lengthen our lives, particularly in later years.

Inflammation is reduced by meditation: Numerous studies on meditation and practices that resemble meditation (yoga, self-hypnosis, methodical structured forms of relaxation, etc.) have also demonstrated anti-inflammatory effects and the suppression of immunological processes that resemble inflammation.

How to Include Meditation in Your Everyday Activities

The best kind of meditation depends on which kind most appeals to the individual among the plethora of available options. I would suggest doing hatha yoga or meditation a few times a week, if not every day, even for fifteen minutes. There are a number of smartphone apps that may guide you through meditation if you have never tried it before and are afraid to enroll in a class. This is especially helpful if you find it difficult to sit still and focus at first. A nutritious diet, frequent exercise, sun protection, getting enough sleep at night, and staying hydrated with water are other important factors to keep in mind if you want to look youthful and vibrant.

Focusing on being acutely aware of your senses and emotions in the present moment, without interpretation or judgment, is the goal of mindfulness meditation. In order to calm the body and mind and lessen stress, mindfulness practices include breathing exercises, guided imagery, and other techniques. Planning, solving problems, fantasizing, or pondering unfavorable or random ideas over extended periods of time can be taxing. It may also increase your likelihood of tension, worry, and depressive symptoms. You may engage with the environment around you and divert your attention from this type of thinking by engaging in mindfulness exercises.

What are the advantages of mindfulness? Numerous clinical trials have examined meditation. Overall, the data point to the benefits of meditation for a number of ailments, such as:

- Intenseness
- Fear and Nervousness
- Depression and pain
- Sleeplessness
- elevated blood pressure, or hypertension

According to a preliminary study, meditation may also be beneficial for those who suffer from fibromyalgia and asthma.

You can experience thoughts and emotions more equitably and acceptingly by practicing meditation. Research has also demonstrated that:

- Increase focus
- Reduce burnout from the workplace
- Boost your sleep
- Boost the management of diabetes

What kinds of workouts promote mindfulness?

Mindfulness can be practiced in a variety of easy ways. Here are a few instances:

Be mindful of this: In a hectic world, taking the time to observe things is difficult. Try to give your surroundings a thorough sensory experience using all of your senses: touch, sound, sight, smell, and taste. For instance, when you eat something you really appreciate, take the time to smell, taste, and savor the dish.

Stay present in the now. Make a conscious effort to approach whatever you do with an open, receptive, and perceptive gaze. Enjoy the small things in life. Accept who you are. As you would a close friend, treat yourself with respect.

Pay attention to how you breathe: Try to sit down, take a deep breath, and close your eyes if you are thinking negatively. Pay attention to how your breath enters and exits your body. Even for a minute, sitting still and breathing might be beneficial. Try more formal mindfulness practices as well, such body scan meditation. Lay down on your back with your arms at your sides and your hands facing upwards. Extend your legs. Slowly and methodically focus your attention on every bodily part, toe to head or head to toe. Become conscious of any feelings, ideas, or sensations connected to every bodily component.

meditation while seated: Place your hands in your lap, your feet flat on the floor, and sit comfortably with your back straight. Pay attention to the inhalation and exhalation of your breath while breathing through your nose. If during your meditation you are interrupted by ideas or physical sensations, acknowledge them and then bring your attention back to your breathing.

Strolling introspection: Choose a space that is 10 to 20 feet long and silent, then start to move slowly. Pay attention to the feelings of standing and the small motions that maintain your equilibrium as you concentrate on the act of walking. Once you've reached the end of your road, turn around and keep moving while paying attention to your feelings.

How often and when should I perform mindfulness exercises?

Depending on the type of mindfulness practice you intend to undertake, yes. Anywhere and at any moment, one can practice basic mindfulness activities. According to research, it's extremely advantageous to use your senses outside. Setting aside time when you can be in a peaceful environment without interruptions is necessary for more structured mindfulness exercises like body scan meditation or seated meditation. Before starting your daily routine, you could decide to perform this kind of exercise first thing in the morning. Try to be mindful every day for approximately half a year. You may eventually discover that mindfulness comes naturally to you. Consider it an undertaking to reestablish and nourish your relationship with yourself.

CHAPTER 7:
Supplements and
Anti-Aging

Dietary supplements can contain a wide range of substances, including vitamins, minerals, herbs, amino acids, enzymes, and other substances that are taken as pills, drinks, gels, capsules, gummies, powder, or as food. The most popular examples are multivitamins, probiotics, herbal supplements, and yes, even protein powders and weight reduction pills fit into this group.

The goal of a supplement is to "supplement" your diet in its entirety by assisting in closing the gap between your typical dietary intake and nutrient requirements. When there is a greater need for certain nutrients, supplements, particularly those containing vitamins and minerals, can be helpful. For instance, there is a greater need for vitamins, minerals, and nutrients—especially folic acid—during pregnancy in order to prevent birth abnormalities. There are certain people who may not be able to obtain enough iron or vitamin D from food alone, or they may have problems with malabsorption. There are, however, a plethora of supplements available, many of which make unsubstantiated health claims. Even if they appear safe, there are a few things to think about before purchasing and utilizing a supplement.

Supplements are not as closely controlled as food and pharmaceuticals, and there is minimal oversight in their case. Before going on sale, they are not required to demonstrate their safety. And the FDA can only act after they are on the market. Despite the use of appropriate manufacturing processes, there are many cases of metals and poisons found in products, as well as significant discrepancies between the product's stated and real levels of active components.

Assertions about the composition and function of supplements do not require scientific evidence to be substantiated.

Certain supplements have the potential to build up to toxic levels and cause medical issues in certain situations. They can also conflict with other medications. All kinds of claims about supplements' ability to "enhance immunity, protect heart health, and improve digestion" are frequently made. However, there is either very little data to back these claims or very few indications for the majority of supplements. For instance, there is conflicting evidence about the heart health advantages of fish oil supplements that include omega-3 fatty acids.

Supplementation may be beneficial for certain populations or people who don't eat fatty fish, but not for others. Furthermore, research on the combination of fish oil supplementation and other medical disorders is even less definitive.

Getting most of our nutrients from food is ultimately the best option. There is, however, a place and a time for supplement use, such as in the case of a deficiency, specific medical conditions, or when evidence of their beneficial effects is available.

Overview of supplements that may support anti-aging

Many of us look to the world of supplements in our never-ending quest to slow down the aging process, viewing them as a kind of mystical elixir. Let's investigate how specific supplements may assist in the pursuit of eternal vitality as we try to solve the secrets underlying these tiny miracles.

1. **Antioxidants:** Antioxidants can be compared to the knights guarding your cells from oxidative stress, the invisible force that accelerates aging. These tiny fighters, which neutralize free radicals and help maintain your cells in fighting shape, are found in vitamins C and E, selenium, and beta-carotene.

2. Omega-3 Fatty Acids: Introducing omega-3 fatty acids, the unsung heroes of aging gracefully and heart health. Supplements containing fish oil are rich in these beneficial fats that maintain the health of your skin, sharpen your mind, and even help reduce inflammation.

3. Consuming Fountain Water: Collagen Supplements: Collagen, the protein that gives your skin its bounce, is becoming more popular in anti-aging. Supplementing with collagen aims to restore the damage caused by aging, which may increase skin moisture and decrease wrinkles. It is akin to taking a sip from the eternal spring.

4. Increasing Cell Energy with Coenzyme Q10 (CoQ10): CoQ10 is essential for the functioning of the mitochondria, which are the powerhouses of the cell. This antioxidant aids in the production of energy by your cells, acting as a kind of energizer. Although further research is required to demonstrate the anti-aging benefits of CoQ10 supplements, they may help you feel more vital.

5. **Resveratrol:** Red grapes and wine contain resveratrol, which is similar to the special guest at the anti-aging celebration. Supplementing with resveratrol may activate genes associated with lifespan, simulating the effects of calorie restriction. The science is still being worked out, but it seems promising.

6. **Vitamin D:** Vitamin D is becoming more important than ever for maintaining healthy bones. Vitamin D pills may be your hidden

weapon for general well being because they've been linked to enhanced immunological response and decreased inflammation.

7. NAD+ Antagonists: Precursors like NR and NMN work to increase NAD+, the VIP of cellular energy. These supplements might improve cellular performance and affect how ageing occurs more elegantly. The early indications are encouraging, but research is still in progress.

Exploring the Supplement Landscape: A Cautionary Note

Although it's tempting to think of a supplement-driven fountain of youth, you should proceed with caution. Since every person's body is an individual universe, what suits one person may not suit another. Speak with a healthcare expert before entering the supplement pool. In addition to providing tailored guidance, they can watch for possible drug or health condition interactions. Supplements are helpful but not the main players when it comes to aging gracefully. Think of them as sidekicks. The traditional remedies of eating well, exercising frequently, and getting enough sleep still shine. Thus, although we delve into the realm of anti-aging supplements, let's remain grounded and realize that the true secret to discovering the mysteries of eternal life is a comprehensive approach.

Consultation with healthcare professionals before adding supplements

Supplements containing vitamins and minerals are examples of supplementary therapies that may interact with prescription drugs and medical procedures. That's the reason it's critical to consult your physician. Seeing a dietician is a smart option if you are told to take vitamin supplements. They can collaborate with your doctor and other medical specialists to provide nutritional advice specific to your needs. It is preferable to take multivitamins at the recommended dietary level rather than high-dose multivitamins or single nutrient supplements if you do need to take a supplement. Recall that whenever you see a medical expert, you should disclose any supplemental medications you are taking, including vitamin and mineral supplements.

CHAPTER 8: Building Healthy Habits

Creating sustainable habits for long-term anti-aging benefits

It's normal to age, but it doesn't have to happen quickly. These anti-aging practices must be followed in order to maintain your immunity, the health of your skin and hair, and your general well-being.

Help Tips:

1. Take an early-morning stroll in the outdoors: Exercise, including walking, can increase energy levels, enhance blood circulation, and stave off chronic conditions like diabetes and cardiovascular diseases.

2. Include ghee in your diet: Its beneficial fats might help to moisturize your skin. It can also be applied externally to ward against wrinkles.

3. Incorporate protein sources into your diet to help you maintain muscle mass, which may help you avoid gaining weight and ward off osteoporosis.

4. Regularly apply sunscreen: You may avoid damaging UV rays and early aging by using sunscreen before going outside.

5. Oil your scalp to nourish your hair: Hair loss might start as you age, but it can be managed with the correct nutrition and care for your stunning locks.

6. Take a collagen supplement for healthy skin: Collagen can have an anti-aging effect on skin and increase skin suppleness and moisture.

7. Eat chia and flax seeds: A healthy gut is linked to good general health, and staying young and fit can be achieved through proper nutrition.

8. Drink lemon or amla juice to strengthen your immunity: Lemon and amla juice are rich in important vitamins and antioxidants that can strengthen your immune system.

9. Steer clear of caffeine: Too much caffeine can affect how well nutrients are absorbed.

The importance of tracking and documenting your anti aging growth

Large-scale changes just don't happen quickly. Observing results from a new skincare regimen may require some time to manifest. In general, it takes 28 to 50 days (depending on your age and skin health) for noticeable benefits to occur as our skin cycle renews. You might believe that your new routine is completely ineffective because these adjustments can occasionally be so subtle.

Because we are constantly exposed to advertisements for "miracle products," you may feel inclined to give up at this crucial point, particularly in this day of immediate gratification, or try something else. But now is the precise moment to exercise patience and keep tabs on your skincare development to see real outcomes and advancements.

Why Monitor Your Development in Skincare?

Selecting the best treatment for your skin type and keeping track of your skincare progress are nearly equally crucial. We're tracking your skincare progress for the following reasons:

- to determine whether the goods you are using are appropriate for the condition of your skin.
- to determine if you need to adjust your routine.
- to know which substances are bad for you and which ones you should use instead.

Ways To Monitor Your Skincare Development

- Preventing the worsening of your skin is the first step in any good skin care routine. The treatment plan then aims to repair and improve the appearance of your skin after that is completed.

- When creating a skin care routine, you should consider your skin type (vata, pitta, or kapha) and any particular treatments your skin may require (dryness, rosacea, acne, anti-aging, etc.). The perfect skincare regimen would include a hydrator, moisturizer, serum, exfoliator, sunscreen, and gentle cleanser based on dosha.

- To ensure that results happen as soon as possible, consistency in use and adherence to a detailed morning and nightly skincare routine are essential.

The following order (to be followed twice a day) should be followed when using them.

Organic Cleanser: Daily Foaming Cleanser for Normal to Dry Skin; Sensitive Skin SBR Cleanser; Oily Skin Pore Perfect Cleanser. Daily, SBR, and Pore Perfect are examples of organic tone/hydrator combinations. All skin types can see noticeable benefits from the Bioscience Peptide Complex in less than 60 days.

Collagen Boost Serum: Provides the skin over 40 with an additional dose of collagen. Restoration moisturizing serum to prevent aging and gently increase collagen in skin under 40. Within 14 to 21 days of use, SBR serum for sensitive, blemished, and rosacea patients produces noticeable benefits (see the interview with a real-life rosacea sufferer to understand how this therapy works).

Taking pictures or a close-up of the troublesome area every seven to fourteen days is the most traditional method of monitoring your skincare progress. To monitor the changes, always utilize the same camera and lighting configurations. The most accurate method of determining the extent of skin healing is to compare these before and after photos.

When should your routine be altered?

You should adjust or switch up your regimen if you still don't see any benefits after two to three cycles, or roughly three months of consistent use.

CONCLUSION

It's not like closing a book when we conclude this guide; rather, it seems like the end of a journey. We looked at dancing with time instead of fighting it as we age in order to maintain our health and happiness.

It has been shown that maintaining good skin care and eating a healthy diet can work like a magic trick to make us feel wonderful. When supplements were first introduced, we discovered that they were more like companions who could support rather than take care of everything. We found that the true magic lies in the ordinary things, such as eating well, getting around, and pausing to enjoy life.

We discussed mindfulness and meditation, which are akin to exercising our minds, in Chapter 7. Not just for eminent yogis, these techniques can improve our mood and even somewhat slow down the aging process. It's as though adopting a happy outlook is a secret weapon against aging.

Here we are at the conclusion, not wanting to go back in time, but realizing that each wrinkle and gray hair has a tale to tell. We are advocating that it's acceptable to have wrinkles on our faces because they are evidence of our shared experiences and laughter.

As we proceed, consider this guidance to be an invitation, a kind recommendation to keep doing the activities that bring us joy. Love the silver hair, accept the wrinkles, and seize every opportunity to be the greatest, happiest versions of ourselves.

Cheers to the path ahead, where there's a chance to enjoy life, remain well, and feel good every single day. With a bright smile and a positive heart, let's toast to becoming older!

GLOSSARY

Aging: is the natural process of aging, marked by a steady deterioration in physical and, in some cases, mental function.

Antioxidants are compounds that protect cells from free radical damage. Vitamin C and vitamin E are common antioxidants.

Balanced Diet: A balanced diet is one that contains a range of foods in the appropriate amounts to provide the nutrients required for good health and energy levels.

Collagen: is a protein that lends shape to the skin, bones, and other tissues. Its production declines with age, resulting in wrinkles and drooping skin.

Exercise: physical activity that boosts strength, flexibility, and overall well-being. Regular exercise is essential for preserving a youthful appearance.

Facial Mask: A skincare product applied to the face for a predetermined amount of time to hydrate, nourish, and cleanse the skin.

Facial Oil: A moisturizing product that nourishes and hydrates the skin, generally incorporating beneficial plant oils.

Free Radicals: are unstable chemicals that can harm cells and contribute to aging and disease. They are neutralized by antioxidants.

Holistic Well-being: A health strategy that takes into account the entire individual, including the physical, mental, and emotional elements.

Meditation: is a practice of concentrated attention and mindfulness that leads to mental clarity, emotional peace, and physical relaxation.

Mindfulness: is the practice of being fully involved in the present moment, which can reduce stress and increase general well-being.

Moisturizer: A skincare product that hydrates and protects the skin, preserving its suppleness and smoothness.

Retinol: a vitamin A derivative that is utilized in skincare products to increase cell turnover and decrease wrinkles.

Serum: A concentrated skincare solution containing active compounds that target specific skin issues, such as aging or hydration.

Skin Care Routine: A daily program of washing, moisturizing, and treating the skin to keep it healthy and attractive.

SPF (Sun Protection Factor): a measurement of a sunscreen's ability to protect the skin against UVB rays. Using SPF protects against UV damage and premature aging.

Stress Management: Techniques and Practices for Regulating Stress Levels and Fostering Mental and Physical Wellness.

Supplements Oral supplements include nutritional elements such as vitamins and minerals to promote general health.

Toner: A skincare product that is applied after cleansing to remove any lingering impurities and prepare the skin for moisturizing and treatment.

Vitamin C Serum: A skincare product containing Vitamin C, which is known for its antioxidant effects as well as its ability to brighten skin and minimize aging signs.

Youthful Skin: Skin that seems healthy, smooth, and lively, often associated with a youthful appearance.

Alpha Hydroxy Acid (AHA): A collection of naturally occurring acids present in foods that are utilized in skincare products for their exfoliating characteristics, which assist in removing dead skin cells and enhancing skin texture.

Bioavailability: The extent and rate with which a substance, such as a nutrient or medication, is absorbed into the bloodstream and available for use by the body.

Botox: Botulinum toxin injections are used as a cosmetic treatment to temporarily paralyze muscles and minimize the appearance of face wrinkles.

Cell Turnover: is the process by which the skin creates new cells while shedding old ones. This process decreases with age, resulting in a bland complexion.

Ceramides: are lipid molecules found in high concentrations within cell membranes in the upper layer of the skin, which are necessary for maintaining the skin's barrier and retaining moisture.

Collagen Peptides: short chains of amino acids derived from collagen that are commonly used as supplements to promote skin, hair, and joint health.

Dental Fillers: are injectable chemicals used to smooth wrinkles, restore volume, and improve facial features.

Elastin: is a protein found in the skin that allows it to return to its former shape after stretching or contracting. As we get older, our elastin levels decrease, which contributes to sagging skin.

Exfoliation: is the removal of dead skin cells from the skin's surface in order to improve texture and encourage cell renewal.

Hyaluronic Acid: is a naturally occurring component in the skin that maintains moisture, keeping it plump and hydrated.

Hyperpigmentation: areas of the skin that grow darker than the surrounding skin due to excessive melanin production, which is frequently caused by sun exposure, inflammation, or hormone fluctuations.

Microdermabrasion: is a minimally invasive technique in which tiny crystals or a diamond-tipped wand exfoliate the skin, decreasing the appearance of fine wrinkles, age spots, and acne scars.

Niacinamide: Also known as Vitamin B3, this skincare ingredient has anti-inflammatory qualities and can improve skin suppleness, strengthen the skin barrier, and even out skin tone.

Oxidative stress: damage to the body produced by an imbalance of free radicals and antioxidants, which can hasten aging and lead to chronic illnesses.

Peptides: Proteins are made up of short chains of amino acids. In skincare, peptides are utilized to increase collagen production and improve skin texture.

Phytochemicals: are chemical molecules produced by plants that have a variety of health benefits, including antioxidant and anti-inflammatory qualities.

Probiotics: are live bacteria that give health advantages, notably to the digestive system, when taken in sufficient quantities. They may also improve skin health when applied topically or consumed orally.

Sirtuins: are a protein family that regulates cellular processes, including aging, by facilitating DNA repair and improving cellular function.

Transepidermal Water Loss (TEWL): The loss of water from the skin to the atmosphere is caused by evaporation. Minimizing TEWL is critical for preserving skin moisture and barrier function.

UVA/UVB Rays: The sun's ultraviolet rays can cause skin damage. UVA rays penetrate deeply, producing long-term damage such as wrinkles; UVB rays cause sunburn and contribute to skin cancer.

Zinc Oxide: A mineral used in sunscreens that may block both UVA and UVB radiation, giving broad-spectrum sun protection.

REVIEW PAGE

Greetings, Reader.

I would like to express my gratitude for taking you on this journey through the Anti Aging Beginners Guide. We really appreciate your time and consideration.

Your opinions count, and as an author, you can never have too much constructive criticism. I would be very appreciative of a review if you liked the book. Your observations can aid in the book's discovery and offer crucial criticism for upcoming releases.

Kindly contemplate expressing your opinions on sites such as [Amazon/Goodreads] or any other preferred venue. In addition to making my day, your frank review will be extremely important in increasing the book's awareness.

Again, thank you for sharing this literary journey. Your help is greatly appreciated.

Sincere greetings
Eve C. Bird